7 Day Introduction to Paleo Fitness

Get Fitter, Get Stronger, Get Healthier in Seven
Days. Move as Nature Intended.

DARRYL EDWARDS

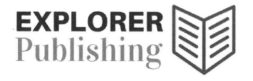

Copyright

Contents

Disclaimer

This book conveys the author's opinions and ideas based on his research, training, and the experiences with his clients.

The material contained within this book is provided for educational and informational purposes only and is not intended as medical, health or other professional services. It should not be used to diagnose or self-treat any illness, metabolic disorder, disease or health problem. You should not consider educational material to be the practice of medicine, physical therapy or personal training.

As with all programmes, techniques and materials related to health, exercise and diet, you must first consult your doctor, physician or health care provider before implementing changes into your lifestyle, following recommendations in this book, or before self-treating any existing conditions.

Responsibility for any results that come from the use of this book lies solely with the reader. The author urges all readers to be aware of their health status and to consult health care professionals before beginning any health, diet or fitness programme.

Introduction

Lack of activity destroys the good condition of every human being, while movement and methodical physical exercise save it and preserve it.
   – Plato

Convenience

With the pace of technological innovation in the past century, movement and physical exertion have become increasingly optional.

Our ancient ancestors chased prey as hunter-gatherers, walked for miles gathering and scavenging food and did whatever they could to avoid predators.

A few hundred years ago we were extensively involved with manual labour on farms and in factories. We spent more time walking, did housework without labour-saving devices and spent no time watching TV or playing video games.

Even though the advantages of physical activity and exercise are extensively researched and documented – which include physical, mental, social and psychological benefits – most of us just don't do enough of it!

Back to Basics

Man's modern environment may have changed dramatically but we can still benefit today by moving as nature intended. One possible solution is to get back to basics and reference the movement patterns of our ancestors; they were naturally lean, robust and healthy based on the activities they had to do daily.

Just as food affects every cell in the body, no organ in the body is unaffected by movement or a lack of it.

The *7 Day Introduction to Paleo Fitness* covers some movement patterns and a workout programme that are geared to the Paleo lifestyle. Enjoy!

Overview

Daily Programming

This workout programme will have you exercising up to six days a week with one day to focus on breathing and mindfulness. That may sound like a lot, especially if you're starting out a workout routine for the first time but this covers various intensities and adequate recovery days and is suitable for beginners as well as for those who want more of a challenge.

Seven Day Programme

This is how we will break down each day:

- **Monday** – is a movement technique day. Here we focus on technique and play around with differing levels of intensity. Instead of an abrupt stop/start of exercises, we want to aim for an uninterrupted flow of movements continuously varied in speed and intensity. Transitioning from one move to the next. Think of this as a slow-paced workout to focus on form with bursts of increased energy and speed.

- **Tuesday and Thursday** – High-Intensity Day. This is where you give it everything you've got! Short but intense. There's a significant amount of evidence that short bursts of high-intensity training, such as sprinting, is more effective for fat-loss than continuous low-intensity aerobic exercise, such as jogging.

- **Wednesday** – is a day to focus on walking. Go for a leisurely stroll and take pleasure in breaking up your usual routine. This is not a power walking exercise but at a slow, almost effortless pace.

- **Friday** – is a day of fun. Taking the opportunity to do something you haven't done before or play around with nostalgia. Stress the fun element rather than your body.

- **Saturday** – focuses on some practical strength and speed training.

- **Sunday** – a breathing exercise to promote relaxation and contemplation based on the achievements of the week.

Enhance The Experience

A few tips to enhance the experience:

1. Go Outside. Take the opportunity to go outside to train. Research tells us about the profound impact that fresh air, grass, trees and colours in the natural environment have on mental health and physical well-being as well as the additional sun exposure that can increase your levels of vitamin D and boost the immune system.

2. Go Barefoot. If you feel comfortable going barefoot (or wish to wear minimalist shoes) for most or all of the activities, then feel free to do so.

3. Be Social. Partner up with friends or family when doing these routines, some of these movements are particularly fun for children too.

4. Focus on your breathing throughout. Don't hold your breath and try to stay as relaxed as possible.

5. Some of the movements you may not be familiar with, so take your time and focus on

your form. Be mindful and consider the importance of the process as well as the goal.

6. Don't feel under pressure to do too much, if a beginner do the lowest number of rounds and the least duration. If you can't complete a workout on a given day or it clashes with something else you have planned, just do so at the first opportunity. No undue pressure required.

7. If you have any questions please feel free to reach out to me via social media – details in the *About The Author* section in the appendix.

Workouts

Movement Monday

Repeat the following movements in sequence for a total of 10, 20 or 30 minutes. Slow, flowing movement. Rest as required.

- *Bear Crawl* x 5 metres
- *Crab Walk* x 5 metres
- *Duck Walk* x 3 metres
- *Kangaroo Jump* x 5 metres

High-Intensity Tuesday

Repeat each exercise for 4, 6 or 8 rounds. Go flat-out at maximum intensity! Rest as required.

- *20 seconds Jump Rope, 10 seconds rest*
- *1 x 30 seconds rest*
- *20 seconds Sprint In Place, 10 seconds rest*
- *1 x 30 seconds rest*
- *20 seconds Air Squat, 10 seconds rest*
- *1 x 30 seconds rest*
- *20 seconds Get-Up/Stand-Up, 10 seconds rest*

Walk Wednesday

Walk for at least 60 minutes in one session.

- Be slow and mindful.

High-Intensity Thursday

Repeat each exercise for 4, 6 or 8 rounds. Go flat-out at maximum intensity! Rest as required.

- 20 seconds *Jump Rope*, 10 seconds rest
- 1 x 30 seconds rest
- 20 seconds *Rabbit Walk*, 10 seconds rest
- 1 x 30 seconds rest
- 20 seconds *Air Squat*, 10 seconds rest
- 1 x 30 seconds rest
- 20 seconds *Dead Hang*, 10 seconds rest

Fun Friday

Friday is reserved for fun. Here are a few suggestions:

- Play tag
- Climb a tree
- Dance to a song you loved as a teenager, on repeat!
- Play catch with the kids
- Walk on some railings

Super Saturday

Repeat each exercise for 4, 6 or 8 rounds. Go flat-out at maximum intensity! Rest as required.

- 100 metre *Sprint* or 20 seconds *Sprint In Place*
- 60 seconds rest
- Push a car for as long as possible (if you don't have a car do a piggy-back carry or run with a heavy loaded backpack)
- 120 seconds rest
- Relax into a 60s Hunter-Gatherer Squat

Relax Sunday

Sunday is a day of relaxation and to congratulate yourself on the efforts you've made this week. Try this simple breathing exercise to reduce blood pressure and to manage stress.

1. Start by clearing your mind and focussing only on your breathing.
2. Feel the air enter your lungs and go out of your lungs
3. Close your mouth and take a deep breath in through the nose for four seconds
4. Hold that breath for eight seconds
5. Breath out through the mouth, slowly and controlled, for eight seconds
6. Repeat steps 1 through 5, four times
7. Finish by breathing normally, but continue to focus on breathing technique

Warm-Ups

Before each workout, perform a *Jump Rope* or *Virtual Jump Rope* for 3-5 minutes.

The Exercises

Air Squat

1. Stand with your feet shoulder-width apart and feet slightly turned out.

2. Bend your knees and sit back as if you were going to sit on a chair, lift your arms up and out to assist with balance and keep a neutral back position.

3. Reverse the movement on the same path as you descended to stand up.

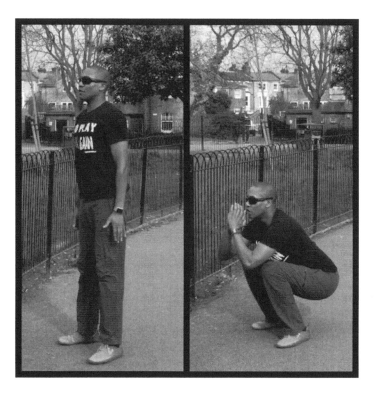

Air Squat

Bear Crawl

1. Start in a low crouched position.

2. Crawl forward on your hands and feet, trying to keep contact with the ground as brief as possible.

3. Avoid using the knees.

4. For an extra challenge, *Bear Crawl* backwards.

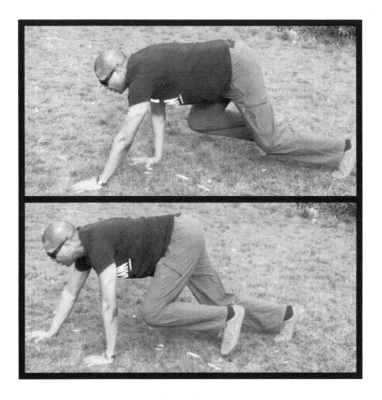

Bear Crawl

Crab Walk

1. From a crouched position, place your hands behind your body and lift your hips so your bottom is off the ground.

2. Keep your palms and feet flat on the ground

3. Start walking forward using hands and feet.

4. For an extra challenge, *Crab Walk* backwards or down the stairs.

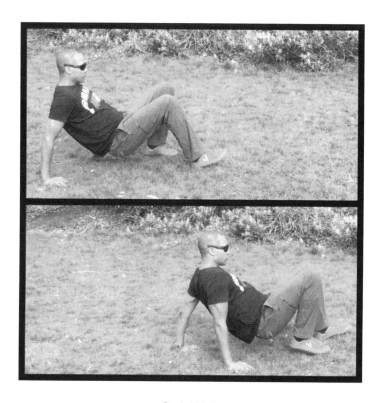

Crab Walk

Dead Hang

1. Hang from a bar or tree branch with your arms in line with your shoulders.

2. Keep your lower body relaxed and don't let your feet touch the ground.

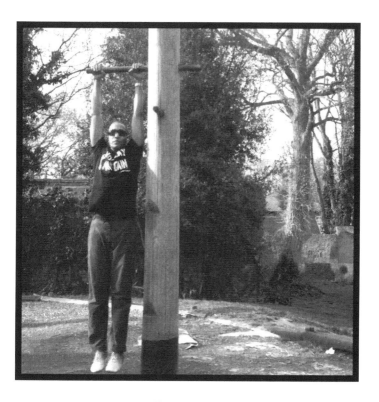

Dead Hang

Duck Walk

1. Start in a low squat position, with your arms resting at your sides with an upright torso.

2. Walk forward and lean slightly forward to stay balanced.

3. For an extra challenge minimise bouncing up and down as you *Duck Walk*.

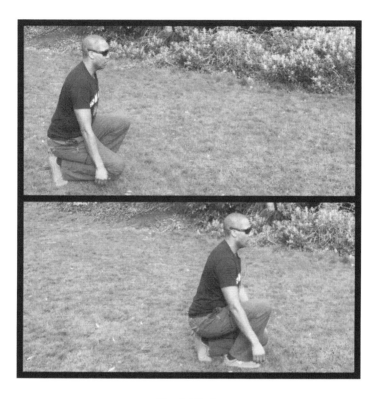

Duck Walk

Get-Up/Stand-Up

1. Stand tall with your arms hanging at your sides.

2. Sit down on the ground. You can use one or both hands for stability.

3. As soon as you sit down entirely, stand straight back up as fast as you can.

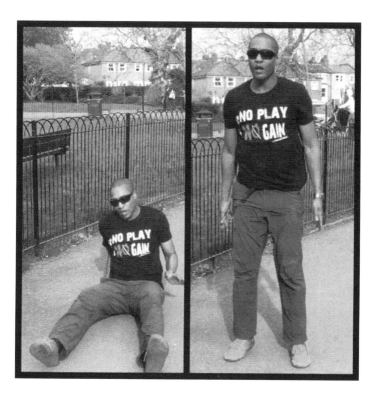

Get-Up/Stand-Up

Hunter-Gatherer Squat

1. Start from a standing position.

2. Sink into a deep squat.

3. Keep your heels flat.

4. Aim to have a relaxed posture in this position.

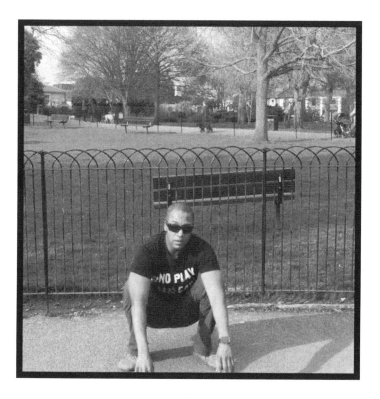

Hunter-Gatherer Squat

Jump Rope (Skipping)

1. Maintain your balance and time your jumps based on the speed of the rope.

2. Focus on being light on your feet.

3. If you can't perform jump rope very well, then just perform the jump rope motion without the rope.

4. For an extra challenge do as many variations of *Jump Rope* as possible.

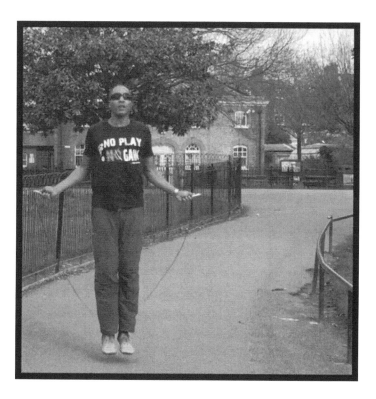

Jump Rope

Kangaroo Jump

1. Stand tall with your feet shoulder-width apart and your arms at the side.

2. Swing your arms behind you to generate power and long jump as far as you can.

3. Land softly on your feet with control and bend your knees to cushion the impact.

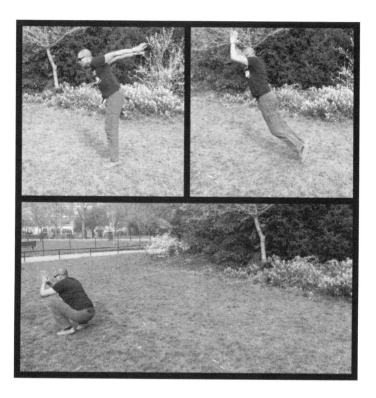

Kangaroo Jump

Rabbit Walk

1. Start in a crouch position.

2. Hop forward onto your arms so your arms take the full weight and your feet are off the floor – tuck your knees into your chest.

3. Drop back to your feet with control.

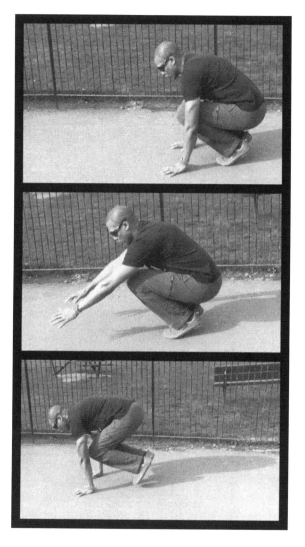

Rabbit Walk

Sprint In Place

1. Sprint on the spot.

2. Stay very light on your feet.

3. For an extra challenge try to raise your knees in front of you above hip height.

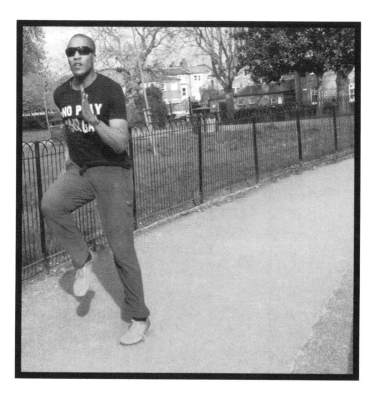

Sprint In Place

Appendix

About The Author

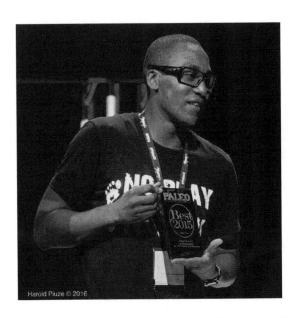

Harold Piuze © 2016

Darryl Edwards, owner of Fitness Explorer Training and Nutrition, founder of HEALTH *Unplugged* and creator of Primal Play. Darryl is an international speaker, certified personal trainer, nutritional therapist, and best-selling author of *Paleo Fitness : Primal Training And Nutrition To Get Lean, Strong And Healthy*, and *Paleo from A to Z. Paleo Fitness* was awarded Best Fitness Book 2015 at the Paleo f(x) awards show. *Paleo from A to Z* was awarded Best Health/Wellness book in the Paleo Magazine's Reader's Choice Award 2016.

Darryl's work has been published in titles such as *Men's Fitness*, *Women's Health*, *Top Santé*, featured on the BBC radio and TV in the UK, and ABC in Australia.

Over ten years ago Darryl embarked on a Paleo approach to well-being when he had no choice but to focus on his health. Back then he was diagnosed with iron-deficiency anaemia, lived with hypertension, had an elevated cardiovascular disease risk profile and 26 per cent body fat, most of it around the middle. He felt weak and lethargic, and suffered from insomnia. He endured low back pain and would often encounter excruciating knee pain when taking part in most activities. He even began to wear knee supports to walk short distances and to walk up stairs.

It didn't take long after focussing on a Paleo lifestyle to reap the benefits and improved health continues to the present day. His body fat now averages 10 per cent, the spare tyre has disappeared, his blood pressure is now in the optimal range, and he is no longer iron-deficient anaemic. His resting heart rate is an *athletic* 38 beats per minute. He's stronger, fitter and healthier now in his forties than at any other period of his life. No more back or knee pain, increased energy levels, and a renewed sense of vitality.

Other biomarkers of health such as cholesterol, blood triglycerides, fasting glucose, vitamin and mineral levels and many other parameters are within normal or optimal ranges, which had not been the case before.

He now advises people on achieving and maintaining a healthy lifestyle amidst the epidemic of obesity and other chronic lifestyle diseases.

Darryl can be found at his health, fitness, nutrition and wellbeing blog, *The Fitness Explorer* (www.theFitnessExplorer.com), where he documents his experience with the Paleo lifestyle and *Primal Play* (www.PrimalPlay.com) where he talks about the importance of living a Play-based lifestyle. He lives in London, England.

Contact Me

Have any questions? Please do not hesitate to get in touch with me on social media or via my websites.

- **Twitter/Instagram**: @FitnessExplorer
- **Facebook**: facebook.com/fitnessexplorer
- **Web**: TheFitnessExplorer.com | PrimalPlay.com

7 Day Introduction to Paleo Fitness

Other Books By Darryl Edwards

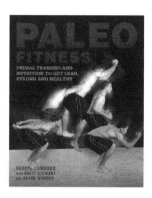

Paleo Fitness: *A Primal Training and Nutrition Program to Get Lean, Strong and Healthy* (Ulysses Press 2013)

- *Paleo Fitness* is packed with step-by-step exercises for an up to 12-week programme, a nutrition primer, a two-week meal plan and delicious, satisfying, healthy recipes. This book shows you how to work out with functional, playful, and primal movements.

- Paleo f(x) Best Fitness Book Award Winner.

- Find out more at: www.PaleoFitnessBook.com.

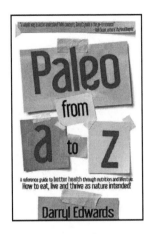

Paleo from A to Z*: A Reference Guide to Better Health Through Nutrition and Lifestyle. How To Eat Live and Thrive as Nature Intended.* (Explorer Publishing 2015)

- The Paleo lifestyle encyclopaedia. *Paleo from A to Z* consists of over 500 topics cutting through the misinformation that surrounds health and nutrition. The listings are in an easy-to-use A-Z format linked to related topics, an appendix of research citations and resources are included too.

- Paleo Magazine Best Health/Wellness Book Winner.

- Find out more at: www.PaleoFromAtoZ.com.

If you like this book please consider writing a review and share your experiences on Amazon, Goodreads, Barnes & Noble, Waterstones, etc.

Amazon Author Page: **http://bit.ly/DarrylEdward**s

Thank you!

27385016R00035

Printed in Great Britain
by Amazon